BEYOND THIRST
H₂O FOR HEALTH

The Science-Backed Benefits of Drinking Water which improve Your Physical & Mental Wellbeing with Every Sip

Blessed Jacobson

Table of Contents

INTRODUCTION

We chug it down after a strenuous workout, reach for it when our throats feel parched, and rely on it for a refreshing pick-me-up on a hot day. Water seems simple, almost mundane. Yet, beneath its seemingly ordinary surface lies a wellspring of life-sustaining power. It's the very foundation of our existence, the elixir that keeps our bodies and minds functioning at their peak. In "H2O for Health: The Science-Backed Benefits of Drinking Water: Improve Your Physical & Mental Wellbeing with Every Sip," we embark on a transformative journey, exploring the remarkable impact of water on our overall well-being.

This book is not just about quenching thirst. It's about unlocking the hidden potential of water, about understanding how this seemingly ordinary molecule can become the catalyst for a healthier, happier you. We'll delve into the fascinating science behind H2O, unveiling its unique properties and the intricate dance it performs within each system of your body. From transporting vital nutrients to lubricating joints, from regulating body temperature to boosting brain function, water plays a starring role in the symphony of life.

Imagine your body as a finely tuned orchestra. Every instrument – your heart, lungs, brain, and muscles needs to function in perfect harmony. But without the conductor, without water, the music falters. Dehydration, even mild, can disrupt this delicate balance, leading to a cascade of negative effects. You might experience fatigue, headaches, difficulty concentrating, and a sluggish metabolism. But by prioritizing hydration, by making water your go-to beverage, you become the conductor, ensuring a smooth and harmonious performance within your body.

But the benefits of water extend far beyond the physical realm. Studies have shown a strong link between proper hydration and improved cognitive function. Imagine sharper focus, enhanced memory, and a clearer mind – all within reach simply by reaching for a glass of water. Additionally, staying hydrated can positively impact your mood, reducing feelings of stress and anxiety and promoting a sense of well-being.

This book is your roadmap to unlocking the transformative power of water. We'll not only explore the science-backed benefits of hydration, but also provide practical strategies to make water an integral part of your daily routine. Learn how to personalize your hydration plan based on your specific needs, discover creative ways to keep your water intake interesting, and overcome common challenges associated with staying hydrated.

"H2O for Health" is more than just a book; it's an invitation. It's an invitation to embark on a journey of self-discovery, to understand the power you hold within your own hands – or rather, in your glass. With each sip of water, you're taking a step towards a healthier, more vibrant you. So, turn the page, raise a glass to your well-being, and prepare to experience the transformative power of H2O for Health. Remember, it all starts with one sip at a time.

THE VITAL ROLE OF WATER

CHAPTER 1:

WHY WATER MATTERS: UNDERSTANDING HYDRATION'S IMPACT ON THE BODY

Water is the most abundant molecule on Earth, freely flowing from our taps and readily available in countless forms. Yet, despite its ubiquity, the true importance of water often goes unrecognized. We often take it for granted, reaching for sugary drinks or neglecting to refill our reusable bottles throughout the day. This chapter delves into the fascinating science behind why water matters, highlighting its profound impact on our physical and mental well-being.

The Foundation of Life: Water's Composition and Remarkable Properties

Water, represented by the simple formula H_2O, is much more than just a combination of hydrogen and oxygen atoms. Its unique structure and properties contribute to its essential role as the foundation of life:

Polarity and Hydrogen Bonding: The uneven distribution of electrons in a water molecule creates a polar character. This, combined with the ability of water molecules to form hydrogen bonds with each other, results in a cohesive force that allows water to resist changes in temperature and form surface tension.

The Universal Solvent: Water's polarity makes it the universal solvent. It can dissolve a wide range of polar molecules like sugars, salts, and proteins, facilitating essential biological reactions within cells.

High Heat Capacity: Water has a remarkable ability to absorb a large amount of heat with a relatively small temperature increase. This property plays a crucial role in regulating Earth's climate and maintaining a stable internal temperature within living organisms.

Beyond Chemistry: Water's Journey Through Your Body

Water makes up roughly 60% of your body weight, making it the most abundant component. It's not just statically present; it's constantly on the move, journeying through your body to support a multitude of functions:

Transportation Network: Water acts as a transport system, carrying essential nutrients, oxygen, and waste products throughout your body via your bloodstream.

Cellular Playground: The majority of cellular processes occur in an aqueous (water-based) environment. Water pave way for these reactions to occur.

Temperature Regulation: When your body temperature rises, you sweat. Water evaporates from your skin, absorbing heat and promoting a cooling effect.

The Symphony of Hydration: Water's Impact on
Every System

From your digestive system to your brain, water plays a vital role in the optimal functioning of every system within your body:

Digestion: Water aids in the breakdown of food and helps move digested material through your intestines, promoting regularity and preventing constipation.

Circulation: Adequate water intake ensures proper blood volume and pressure, allowing for efficient blood flow and delivery of oxygen and nutrients to your organs.

Brain Function: Even mild dehydration can impair cognitive function, memory, and focus. Water ensures your brain cells have the resources they need to function optimally.

Musculoskeletal System: Water lubricates joints, prevents muscle stiffness and soreness, and helps deliver nutrients to your muscles for optimal performance and recovery.

Skin Health: Hydrated skin has a healthy glow and elasticity. Dehydration can lead to dry, flaky skin and exacerbate wrinkles.

The Dehydration Drain: Consequences of Neglecting Water Needs

While thirst serves as a basic indicator of dehydration, neglecting your water needs can have significant consequences well before you experience thirst:

- Reduced Physical Performance: Dehydration diminishes your endurance and can lead to fatigue, hindering your ability to perform at your best during exercise.
- Headaches: Dehydration is a frequent culprit behind headaches, impacting your focus and productivity.
- Kidney Function: Water helps flush out waste products from your kidneys. Dehydration can put extra strain on your kidneys and increase the risk of kidney stones.
- Mood Swings and Irritability: Dehydration can negatively impact your mood, leading to feelings of irritability and fatigue.

- Impaired Cognitive Function: Even mild dehydration can affect your focus, concentration, and memory.

The Importance of Individualized Hydration:

Several factors influence your daily water requirements:

- The Size of your Body: Individuals with larger body size require generally require more water than smaller individuals.
- Activity Level: Physical activity increases your body's water needs. The more you sweat, the more water you need to replenish.
- Climate: Hot and humid climates increase your body's water loss through sweat, requiring increased water intake.
- Overall Health: Certain health conditions may necessitate adjustments in water intake.

Beyond Plain Water: Optimizing Your Hydration Strategy

While water is the foundation of optimal hydration, there are additional strategies to ensure you're meeting your body's water needs:

Food Choices: Many fruits and vegetables have a high water content. Incorporating them into your diet can contribute significantly to your daily hydration. Think watermelon, cucumber, celery, and leafy greens.

Listen to Your Thirst: While not a foolproof indicator, thirst is your body's natural signal that it needs water. Don't wait until you're parched to reach for a drink.

Carry a Reusable Water Bottle: Having a water bottle readily available throughout the day serves as a constant reminder to sip water and stay hydrated.

Flavor Boosters: For some, plain water can become monotonous. Adding slices of fruits, herbs, or vegetables to your water can enhance the flavor and encourage water intake.

Hydration Apps and Reminders: There are numerous hydration apps and trackers available to help you monitor your water intake and set reminders to sip water throughout the day.

Breaking the Soda Habit and Choosing Water-Wisely

Sugary drinks and sodas may provide a temporary thirst quench, but they can also contribute to dehydration and a host of health problems. Here's why water is the clear winner:

Empty Calories and Added Sugars: Sugary drinks are packed with empty calories and added sugars, contributing to weight gain and other health concerns. Water, on the other hand, has zero calories and is essential for maintaining a healthy weight.

Increased Urination: The diuretic effect of caffeine and certain artificial ingredients in sugary drinks can lead to increased urination, potentially leading to dehydration.

Long-Term Health Risks: Excessive consumption of sugary drinks is linked to an increased risk of chronic health problems like diabetes, heart disease, and certain cancers.

The Future of Hydration: Personalized Approaches and Emerging Technologies

The field of hydration science is constantly evolving. Here are idea into what the future might hold:

Personalized Hydration Recommendations: Technological advancements may lead to the development of personalized hydration plans based on factors like individual physiology, activity level, and environmental conditions.

Smart Hydration Bottles and Wearable: Smart water bottles and wearable devices with hydration tracking capabilities may become even more sophisticated, providing real-time feedback and personalized hydration reminders.

Focus on Hydration in Healthcare: As the understanding of the impact of hydration on health continues to grow, healthcare providers may place a greater emphasis on personalized hydration counseling and education.

Water is the cornerstone of health and well-being. By understanding the science behind why water matters and adopting practical strategies to stay hydrated, you can embark on a life-long journey towards optimal health, improved physical performance, and a sharper, more focused mind. Remember, every sip counts. Make water your go-to beverage and prioritize hydration throughout the day. Your body will thank you for it!

The next chapter will delve deeper into the fascinating science of water, exploring its unique properties and the intricate role it plays within each system of your body.

CHAPTER 2:

UNVEILING THE MAGIC OF H2O: A DEEPER DIVE INTO WATER'S COMPOSITION AND REMARKABLE PROPERTIES

Water, the seemingly simple molecule represented by H2O, holds the key to life on Earth. Beyond quenching thirst, water possesses unique properties that make it essential for a wide range of biological and chemical processes. In this chapter, we'll delve deeper into the fascinating science of water, exploring its composition, unique properties, and its role as the foundation of life.

Unpacking the Molecule: The Building Blocks of H2O

Water is a deceptively simple molecule, consisting of two hydrogen atoms bonded to a single oxygen atom. However, the arrangement of these atoms and the nature of the bonds they share contribute to water's remarkable properties.

Polar Covalent Bonding: The sharing of electrons between the oxygen and hydrogen atoms in water is unequal. Oxygen has a higher electronegativity, attracting electrons more strongly, resulting in a polar covalent bond. This uneven distribution of charge creates a slight positive charge on the hydrogen ends and a slight negative charge on the oxygen end, giving water its polar character.

Hydrogen Bonding: The Architect of Water's Structure

The polar nature of water molecules leads to a unique phenomenon – hydrogen bonding. The positively charged hydrogen end of one water molecule is attracted to the negatively charged oxygen end of another water molecule, forming a weak but crucial bond. Hydrogen bonding creates a three-dimensional network that gives water several of its distinctive properties:

High Cohesion: Hydrogen bonding allows water molecules to stick to each other, creating a high degree of cohesion. This property is responsible for surface tension, the force that allows water to form droplets and bead on surfaces.

Adhesion: Hydrogen bonding also allows water molecules to adhere to other polar molecules. This is essential for water's interaction with biological molecules like proteins and carbohydrates, forming the foundation of life processes.

Another fascinating property of water is its unique density behavior. Unlike most substances, water reaches its highest density at 4°C. As the temperature decreases further, water expands and becomes less dense, which is why ice floats in water. This anomaly is crucial for life on Earth:

Life under Ice: If ice were denser than liquid water, it would sink to the bottom of lakes and oceans, eventually freezing all bodies of water. The unique density behavior of water allows for the formation of ice on top, creating a layer of insulation that protects life beneath the frozen surface.

The Universal Solvent: Water's Remarkable Ability to Dissolve

Water is often referred to as the "universal solvent" due to its exceptional ability to dissolve a wide range of substances. This property is also a consequence of its polar nature and hydrogen bonding:

Solvating Ionic Compounds: Ionic compounds, such as table salt ($NaCl$), dissociate in water. The polar water molecules surround the charged ions (Na^+ and Cl^-), weakening the attraction between them and allowing the ions to dissolve.

Hydration of Polar Molecules: Water molecules can also form hydrogen bonds with polar molecules like sugars and proteins. This "hydration" process allows these molecules to dissolve in water and participate in essential biological reactions.

Water's Role in Chemical Reactions: A Catalyst for Change

Water is not just a passive participant in biological processes; it also acts as a catalyst, accelerating the rate of chemical reactions within cells. This occurs because:

Hydrolysis Reactions: Water molecules can break down larger molecules through a process called hydrolysis. This is crucial for digestion and the breakdown of nutrients in the body.

Acid-Base Reactions: Water acts as both an acid and a base, depending on the situation. This allows it to participate in acid-base reactions, which are essential for maintaining a stable pH level within cells.

The Heat Capacity Conundrum: Water's Role in Temperature Regulation

Water has a high heat capacity, meaning it can absorb a significant amount of heat with a relatively small increase in temperature. This property plays a vital role in regulating Earth's climate and maintaining a stable internal temperature in living organisms:

Oceanic Heat Buffer: The vast oceans absorb a large amount of the sun's heat, acting as a buffer and preventing drastic temperature fluctuations on Earth.

Temperature Regulation in Living Beings: Water's high heat capacity allows organisms to maintain a relatively constant internal temperature, even when the external environment changes. Sweating, a process facilitated by water evaporation, also helps cool the body down.

Acidity and pH: The Delicate Balance in Water

Water itself is a weak electrolyte, meaning it can dissociate into a small degree of hydrogen (H+) and hydroxide (OH-) ions.

The concentration of these ions determines the pH of a solution, a measure of acidity or alkalinity. Understanding pH is crucial for understanding water's role in various biological processes:

The pH Scale: Solutions with a pH lower than 7 are acidic (higher concentration of H+ ions), while solutions with a pH higher than 7 are basic (higher concentration of OH- ions).

Maintaining a Stable pH: The body tightly regulates its internal pH within a narrow range, typically between 7.35 and 7.45. Water plays a crucial role in this regulation by acting as a buffer system, neutralizing small changes in acid or base concentration.

The Intricacy of Water's Chemical Equilibria

The dissociation of water molecules into H+ and OH- ions is an ongoing equilibrium process. This means the forward and backward reactions (dissociation and recombination) occur simultaneously:

Le Chatelier's Principle: According to Le Chatelier's principle, a system at equilibrium will respond to changes by shifting the equilibrium position to minimize the effect of the change. Understanding this principle is essential for comprehending how the body maintains a stable pH.

Water's Role in Biological Processes: The Foundation of Life

From transporting nutrients to facilitating cellular reactions, water plays a vital role in countless biological processes:

Transportation: Water serves as a transport medium for essential nutrients, oxygen, and waste products throughout the body. Blood, for example, is largely composed of water.

Cellular Reactions: Many biochemical reactions within cells occur in an aqueous (water-based) environment. Water acts as a solvent, allowing reactants to interact and facilitating these reactions.

Lubrication: Water is a lubricant for joints and other tissues, reducing friction and promoting smooth movement.

Regulation: Water plays a role in regulating body temperature, blood pressure, and other vital functions.

Water, in its apparent simplicity, holds the key to life on Earth. Its unique properties – from hydrogen bonding to its high heat capacity – make it essential for a wide range of biological and chemical processes. Understanding the science behind water unlocks a deeper appreciation for its vital role in our own health and the delicate balance of life on our planet.

In the next chapter, we'll explore how water's influence extends beyond its chemical properties, impacting every system within our bodies and contributing to our overall well-being.

CHAPTER 3:

BEYOND QUENCHING THIRST: HOW WATER AFFECTS EVERY SYSTEM IN YOUR BODY

Water. It's the simplest, most overlooked substance we consume, yet it plays a vital role in every system within our bodies. It's more than just a thirst quencher; it's the foundation for optimal health and well-being. In this chapter, we'll embark on a fascinating journey through the human body, exploring the diverse and far-reaching effects of water on each of our vital systems.

The Digestive Symphony: Water as a Conductor of Smooth Functioning

Imagine your digestive system as an intricate orchestra. Water acts as the conductor, ensuring all the instruments – from the esophagus to the intestines – function smoothly. Here's how:

Breakdown and Absorption of Nutrients: Water is essential for breaking down food into its component parts, making it easier for your body to absorb essential nutrients. Constipation and other digestive problem can occur as a result of Dehydration.

Regulation of Bowel Movements: Water keeps things moving by softening stool and promoting regular bowel movements. Dehydration can contribute to constipation and hemorrhoids.

Aiding in Liver Function: The liver plays a crucial role in detoxification. Water helps the liver flush out waste products and toxins, keeping your digestive system functioning optimally.

The Circulatory System: Water, the Essential Flow

Imagine of your circulatory system as a numerous network of rivers and streams. Water is the lifeblood that keeps this network flowing efficiently:

Blood Volume and Pressure Regulation: Water makes up a significant portion of your blood volume. Adequate hydration ensures proper blood pressure and circulation, delivering oxygen and nutrients throughout your body.

Transport of Essential Components: Water serves as a transport system for essential components like blood cells, hormones, and electrolytes. These components rely on water to reach their destinations and perform their vital functions.

Regulation of Body Temperature: When you sweat, your body releases heat through evaporation. Water is essential for sweating, which helps maintain a healthy body temperature.

The Respiratory Symphony: Water for Smooth Breathing

Your respiratory system, the orchestra of your breath, also relies on water for optimal performance:

Moistening Air Passages: Water helps keep your airways moist, allowing for smooth passage of air during inhalation and exhalation. Dehydration can lead to dry, irritated airways, making breathing uncomfortable.

Mucus Production: Your body produces mucus to trap dust and irritants in your airways. Water helps maintain the proper consistency of mucus, allowing it to function effectively.

Defense against Respiratory Infections: Proper hydration strengthens your body's natural defenses, helping to fight off respiratory infections like the common cold.

The Musculoskeletal System: Water, the Lubricant for Movement

Your musculoskeletal system, the complex machinery that allows you to move, thrives on hydration:

Lubrication of Joints: Water acts as a lubricant for your joints, ensuring smooth, pain-free movement. Joint pain and stiffness can be as result of dehydration.

Delivery of Nutrients to Muscles: Water transports essential nutrients to your muscles, providing them with the fuel they need to function and recover after exercise.

Regulation of Body Temperature: As mentioned earlier, water plays a role in regulating body temperature. This is crucial for muscles, as proper temperature is essential for optimal performance and preventing overheating.

The Nervous System: Water, the Conductor of Electrical Signals

Your nervous system, the electrical network that controls all bodily functions, relies heavily on water:

Transmission of Nerve Impulses: Water is essential for the transmission of nerve impulses throughout your body. Dehydration can disrupt this process, leading to impaired coordination, confusion, and fatigue.

Brain Function and Cognitive Performance: As discussed in the next chapter, water plays a vital role in brain function. Dehydration can negatively impact cognitive performance, focus, and memory.

Mood Regulation: There's a growing body of research suggesting that dehydration can contribute to mood swings and irritability. Staying hydrated can help maintain emotional balance.

The Integumentary System: Water for a Healthy Glow

Your integumentary system, the largest organ of your body (comprising your skin, hair, and nails), benefits from proper hydration:

Skin Hydration and Elasticity: Water is essential for plumping and hydrating your skin cells, giving you a healthy, youthful appearance. Dehydration can lead to dry, flaky skin and exacerbate wrinkles.

Temperature Regulation: Your skin plays a role in regulating body temperature. Water helps with sweating, a key mechanism for keeping you cool.

Nutrient Delivery and Waste Removal: Water helps transport nutrients to your skin cells and flushes out waste products, promoting overall skin health.

As we've explored, water acts as a conductor within each system of your body, ensuring smooth operation and optimal function. Dehydration, on the other hand, disrupts this delicate symphony, leading to a cascade of negative effects. By prioritizing hydration, you're essentially investing in the health and well-being of your entire being.

While water is the foundation of optimal hydration, there are other lifestyle choices that can support your body's water needs:

A Balanced Diet: Fruits and vegetables are naturally high in water content. Incorporating them into your diet can contribute significantly to your daily hydration needs.

Electrolytes for Replenishment: Electrolytes, like sodium and potassium, play a role in fluid balance and muscle function. Consider electrolyte-rich foods like fruits and vegetables, or consult a healthcare professional regarding electrolyte supplements if needed, particularly for high-intensity exercise.

Limiting Diuretics: Certain beverages like coffee and alcohol can have a diuretic effect, increasing urination and potentially leading to dehydration. Be mindful of your intake and prioritize water.

Quality Sleep: When you're well-rested, your body functions more efficiently, including regulating water balance. Aim for 7-8 hours of quality sleep each night.

The Power of Consistency: Building Sustainable Hydration Habits

Developing sustainable hydration habits is key to reaping the long-term benefits of proper water intake. Here are some tips:

Find a Water Bottle You Love: Invest in a reusable water bottle that you find aesthetically pleasing and convenient to carry with you throughout the day.

Set Hydration Reminders: Use apps, alarms, or sticky notes to remind yourself to sip water at regular intervals.

Infuse Your Water for Flavor: Add slices of fruits, herbs, or vegetables to your water for a refreshing and flavorful twist.

Pair Water with Meals and Snacks: Make water your go-to beverage at mealtimes and in between snacks.

Celebrate Your Progress: Acknowledge your efforts, no matter how small. Seeing your progress can be a great motivator to stay on track.

Hydration: A Journey for a Healthier You

Hydration is a lifelong journey, not a destination. By incorporating these strategies and making water an essential part of your daily routine, you'll be well on your way to experiencing the transformative power of water on your overall health and well-being. Remember, every sip counts. So, raise a glass to a future filled with vitality, optimal function, and a body that thrives on the simple yet powerful act of staying hydrated!

UNVEILING THE BENEFITS OF HYDRATION

CHAPTER 4:

BRAINPOWER BOOST: HOW WATER ENHANCES COGNITIVE FUNCTION AND MOOD

Our brains are the command centers of our existence, orchestrating everything from complex thoughts to basic movements. They are also incredibly thirsty organs, requiring a steady supply of water to function optimally. In this chapter, we'll delve into the fascinating science behind water's impact on cognitive function and mood, revealing how proper hydration can be the key to unlocking a sharper, more focused you.

The human brain is roughly 73% water. This seemingly simple fact translates to a profound truth – water is fundamental for optimal brain function. Here's how:

Hydration for Optimal Electrical Activity: The brain relies on electrical signals to transmit information between neurons. Dehydration can disrupt these electrical signals, leading to impaired cognitive function.

Enhanced Blood Flow: Water is crucial for maintaining healthy blood flow, which delivers oxygen and essential nutrients to the brain cells, fueling their activity.

Sharpening Focus and Concentration: Mild dehydration can lead to decreased focus, attention span, and difficulty concentrating. Staying hydrated ensures your brain has the resources it needs to operate at its peak.

Improved Memory Consolidation: Water plays a role in memory consolidation, the process by which short-term memories are converted into long-term storage. Dehydration can impair this process, affecting your ability to learn and retain information.

The Dehydration Drain: Consequences for Cognitive Function

Even mild dehydration (around 2% of body weight) can have a noticeable impact on cognitive function:

Reduced Alertness and Mental Fatigue: Dehydration can make you feel sluggish and less alert. Simple tasks might feel more challenging, and you might find it harder to stay focused throughout the day.

Impaired Decision-Making: Dehydration can cloud your judgment and hinder your ability to make clear decisions.

Decreased Creativity and Problem-Solving Skills: Staying hydrated ensures your brain has the resources it needs for creative thinking and problem-solving. Dehydration can stifle these abilities.

Headaches: Dehydration is a frequent culprit behind headaches, further contributing to cognitive difficulties.

Water's influence extends beyond cognitive function, impacting your mood and overall well-being:

Improved Mood and Reduced Irritability: Dehydration can contribute to irritability, frustration, and even anxiety. Staying hydrated can help maintain a positive mood and emotional balance.

Enhanced Energy Levels: When your brain is properly hydrated, it operates more efficiently, leading to increased energy levels and a sense of vitality.

Reduced Stress and Improved Coping Mechanisms: Dehydration can exacerbate stress. Proper hydration can help your body cope with stress more effectively.

Better Sleep Quality: Dehydration can disrupt sleep patterns. Adequate hydration promotes quality sleep, which is crucial for both cognitive function and emotional well-being.

Hydration Strategies for a Sharper, Happier You

Now that you understand the science, let's explore practical strategies to optimize your hydration for enhanced cognitive function and mood:

Listen to Your Thirst Cues: While the "eight glasses a day" rule is a general guideline, individual needs vary. Pay attention to your thirst cues – aim for clear urine and avoid feeling excessively thirsty.

Make Water Your Go-To Beverage: Swap sugary drinks, sodas, and excessive coffee for water. Opt for sparkling water infused with fruits or herbs for a touch of flavor if plain water feels monotonous.

Carry a Reusable Water Bottle: Having a water bottle readily available serves as a constant reminder to sip water throughout the day.

Eat Water-Rich Foods: Fruits and vegetables like watermelon, cucumber, and celery have a high water content, contributing to your daily hydration needs.

Set Hydration Reminders: Use apps or alarms to remind yourself to sip water throughout the day.

While water is the foundation of optimal hydration, there are other things you can do to support cognitive function and mood:

A Balanced Diet: Nourish your brain with a healthy diet rich in fruits, vegetables, whole grains, and lean protein. These foods provide essential nutrients that fuel brain function.

Regular Exercise: Physical activity increases blood flow to the brain, promoting the delivery of oxygen and nutrients.

Quality Sleep: 7-8 hours of quality sleep each night should be your target. Sleep is essential for memory consolidation and cognitive function.

Stress Management Techniques: Chronic stress can negatively impact your brain. Techniques like meditation, yoga, or deep breathing can help manage stress and promote a calmer mind-state.

By embracing proper hydration and incorporating these holistic strategies, you can embark on a journey towards a sharper, more focused you. Remember, consistency is key. Don't expect overnight results; focus on developing sustainable habits that make staying hydrated second nature. Celebrate small victories, like remembering to carry your water bottle, and witness the cumulative impact on your cognitive function and overall well-being.

Here are some additional tips to maximize the cognitive benefits of staying hydrated:

Start Your Day with Water: Drinking a glass of water first thing in the morning jumpstarts your hydration and helps clear your mind for the day ahead.

Pair Water with Meals and Snacks: Make water your beverage of choice at mealtimes and in between snacks. This ensures a steady flow of hydration throughout the day.

Hydrate before Important Tasks: Whether it's a presentation, a challenging exam, or a complex problem to solve, ensure you're well-hydrated beforehand. Proper hydration can enhance your focus and cognitive abilities.

Track Your Progress: Use a hydration tracking app or a simple log to monitor your water intake. Seeing your progress can be a motivator to stay on track.

The good news is that good hydration habits are relatively easy to form. By incorporating these strategies into your daily routine, you'll be well on your way to automatic hydration, where staying hydrated becomes a natural and effortless part of your day.

Just as a well-tuned orchestra requires each instrument to function optimally, our brains rely on a symphony of factors for peak performance. Water acts as the conductor of this symphony, ensuring that all the elements – nutrients, oxygen, and electrical signals – flow smoothly, leading to enhanced cognitive function, improved mood, and well-being in every aspect of your life.

So, raise a glass to a future filled with sharper focus, enhanced decision-making, a brighter mood, and a brain that thrives on the power of hydration!

CHAPTER 5:

PHYSICAL PERFORMANCE PEAK: OPTIMIZING ENERGY LEVELS AND EXERCISE RECOVERY

For athletes, pushing their limits is a constant pursuit. Whether you're a seasoned marathoner or a weekend warrior striving for personal bests, optimizing performance and recovery are paramount. In this chapter, we'll delve into the science behind water's crucial role in both, highlighting how proper hydration can elevate your game and accelerate your recovery journey.

Every aspect of athletic performance, from muscular function to cognitive focus, relies heavily on water. Here's how proper hydration fuels your athletic endeavors:

Enhanced Muscle Function: Water acts as a lubricant for your joints and muscles, ensuring smooth movement and reducing the risk of friction-related injuries. Muscle cramps, fatigue, and decreased power output can be as result of proper hydration.

Temperature Regulation: During exercise, your body generates heat. Water plays a vital role in sweating, a natural cooling mechanism that helps maintain optimal body temperature for peak performance.

Improved Cognitive Performance: Even mild dehydration can impair cognitive function, affecting focus, reaction time, and decision-making. Staying hydrated ensures your brain operates at its best during training and competition.

Delivery of Nutrients and Oxygen: Water transports essential nutrients and oxygen to your working muscles, providing them with the fuel they need to function optimally and generate energy.

The Dehydration Drain: Consequences for Performance

Dehydration, even at a minor level (around 2% of body weight), can significantly impact athletic performance:

Reduced Endurance: Dehydration decreases your ability to sustain high-intensity exercise for extended periods.

Increased Fatigue: Muscle fatigue sets in earlier when your body is dehydrated, hindering your ability to push yourself.

Impaired Concentration: As mentioned earlier, dehydration can impact focus and reaction time, potentially leading to mistakes during training or competition.

Increased Risk of Heatstroke: Severe dehydration can lead to heatstroke, a dangerous condition requiring immediate medical attention.

Beyond Performance: Water's Role in Recovery

Hydration doesn't end after your workout. Water plays a crucial role in the recovery process:

Aiding Muscle Repair: Water helps flush out waste products produced by exercise, such as lactic acid, which can contribute to muscle soreness.

Replenishing Fluids and Electrolytes: Sweating depletes electrolytes like sodium and potassium. Water helps replenish these essential minerals, aiding in proper muscle function and nerve transmission.

Promoting Tissue Repair: Water is essential for transporting nutrients to your muscles, which are crucial for rebuilding and repairing tissues after exercise.

Improving Sleep Quality: Dehydration can disrupt sleep patterns. Adequate hydration promotes better sleep, which is vital for optimal recovery.

Hydration Strategies for Peak Performance and Recovery

Now that you understand the science, let's explore practical strategies to optimize your hydration for peak performance and recovery:

Individualize Your Needs: Fluid needs vary based on factors like body size, activity level, and climate. Consider consulting a nutritionist to determine your personalized hydration requirements.

Hydrate Before, During and After Exercise: Drink water 1-2 hours before your workout to pre-hydrate. Aim for small sips of water every 15-20 minutes during exercise. Continue to rehydrate after your workout to replenish fluids lost through sweat.

Monitor Your Urine Color: Pale yellow urine indicates adequate hydration. Dark yellow urine suggests dehydration.

Invest in a Reusable Water Bottle: Having a water bottle with you at all times serves as a constant reminder to sip water throughout the day.

Electrolytes for Extended Exercise: For long-duration or high-intensity workouts, consider electrolyte-containing beverages to replenish electrolytes lost through sweat.

While water is the foundation of optimal hydration, athletes may also benefit from incorporating other strategies:

Focus on a Balanced Diet: A diet rich in fruits, vegetables, and whole grains provides your body with essential nutrients and additional fluids.

Prioritize Sleep: 7-8 hours of quality sleep each night should always be your target. Sleep allows your body to repair and rebuild tissues, and dehydration can disrupt sleep patterns.

Post-Workout Recovery Techniques: Techniques like foam rolling, stretching, and massage can further enhance recovery by promoting blood flow and reducing muscle soreness.

Listen to Your Body: Pay attention to your thirst cues and adjust your water intake accordingly. Pushing yourself to drink excessive amounts of water can be counterproductive.

By embracing proper hydration and incorporating these strategies into your training regimen, you can empower your body to perform at its peak and accelerate your recovery journey. Remember, consistency is key. Don't expect immediate results; focus on developing sustainable hydration habits that become second nature. Celebrate your progress, no matter how small, and enjoy the empowering sense of control that comes from fueling your body with its most essential ingredient – water.

For serious athletes and individuals participating in endurance events, additional considerations might be necessary:

Sweat Testing: A sweat test can analyze your individual electrolyte losses through sweat, helping you tailor your electrolyte replacement strategy during exercise.

Sports Drinks vs. Electrolyte Tablets: Choose sports drinks or electrolyte tablets based on your needs. Sports drinks can be beneficial for shorter, high-intensity workouts, while electrolyte tablets might be more suitable for longer durations where concentrated sugar intake isn't ideal.

Monitoring Hydration Status with Technology: Wearable hydration trackers can estimate sweat loss and provide real-time feedback to ensure you're staying adequately hydrated.

Hydration and Mental Toughness: A Synergistic Relationship

Proper hydration isn't just about physical performance. It also contributes to mental toughness, a crucial component of athletic success. Here's how:

Enhanced Focus and Concentration: As discussed earlier, dehydration can impair cognitive function, making it difficult to stay focused and make critical decisions during training or competition.

Improved Mood and Motivation: Dehydration can contribute to fatigue and irritability. Staying hydrated can help maintain a positive mood and enhance motivation to push yourself further.

Increased Resilience: Hydration supports your body's ability to handle physical and mental stress, allowing you to persevere through challenging workouts and competitions.

By prioritizing hydration, you're essentially conducting a symphony within your body, optimizing every system for peak performance and recovery. Remember, water is the conductor, orchestrating the flow of nutrients, oxygen, and waste products. Listen to your body's cues, personalize your hydration strategies, and witness the transformative power of water in propelling you towards your athletic goals.

So, raise a glass to a future of peak performance, accelerated recovery, and a mind and body empowered by the simple yet powerful act of staying hydrated!

CHAPTER 6:

WEIGHT MANAGEMENT ALLY: WATER'S ROLE IN APPETITE CONTROL AND METABOLISM

In the ongoing battle against unwanted pounds, water often gets relegated to the sidelines. However, the truth is, water plays a vital role in weight management, acting as a powerful ally in your journey towards a healthier you. This chapter delves into the science behind how water can support your weight management goals by influencing appetite control and metabolism.

Dehydration can often be mistaken for hunger. When your body is thirsty, it can send signals that mimic hunger pangs. Here's how water helps curb your appetite:

Filling Up on Fewer Calories: Water has zero calories, yet it can create a feeling of fullness in your stomach. Drinking water before meals can help you consume fewer calories overall.

Reduced Ghrelin, the Hunger Hormone: Studies suggest that dehydration can lead to increased levels of ghrelin, the hormone that stimulates appetite. Adequate water intake helps regulate ghrelin levels, keeping hunger pangs in check.

Increased Satiety Hormones: Water consumption can promote the release of hormones like leptin, which signal feelings of fullness to your brain. This can help you feel satisfied for longer periods, reducing cravings between meals.

Beyond Appetite Control: Water's Metabolic Boost

Water plays a crucial role in various bodily functions that impact metabolism, the rate at which your body burns calories. Here's how:

Enhanced Digestion and Nutrient Absorption: Water is essential for proper digestion and nutrient absorption. Dehydration can slow down digestion, leading to bloating and a sluggish metabolism.

Transportation of Nutrients: Water acts as a transport system, carrying essential nutrients to your cells, where they can be used for energy production and various metabolic processes.

Regulation of Body Temperature: Maintaining a healthy body temperature is crucial for optimal metabolism. Water helps regulate body temperature through sweating, ensuring your body functions efficiently.

The Science of Water-Induced Thermogenesis

While the calorie-burning effect of water is often debated, there's evidence to suggest that water can induce thermogenesis, the process by which your body burns calories to generate heat. Studies have shown that cold water consumption can increase energy expenditure slightly, although the exact mechanisms are still being explored.

Hydration Strategies for Successful Weight Management

Let's explore practical strategies to leverage water's power for weight management:

Drink Water Before Meals: Aim for a glass of water 30 minutes before each meal. This can help you feel fuller and consume fewer calories during your meal.

Carry a Reusable Water Bottle: Having a water bottle with you throughout the day serves as a constant reminder to sip water and stay hydrated.

Set Hydration Reminders: Use apps or alarms to remind yourself to drink water at regular intervals.

Flavor up Your Water: If plain water feels monotonous, add slices of fruits, herbs, or vegetables for a refreshing and flavorful twist.

Choose Water Over Sugary Drinks: Swap sugary sodas, juices, and sports drinks for water. These beverages are loaded with calories and can sabotage your weight management efforts.

Pair Water with Exercise: Drinking water before, during, and after exercise is essential for hydration and can also help boost your metabolism.

While water is a powerful tool for weight management, it's important to remember that it's not a magic bullet. A sustainable weight loss approach requires a combination of healthy eating habits, regular exercise, and adequate sleep.

Focus on Whole, Unprocessed Foods: Base your diet on whole, unprocessed foods like fruits, vegetables, and whole grains. These foods are naturally filling and provide essential nutrients for your body.

Embrace Portion Control: Practice mindful eating and pay attention to portion sizes. Avoid talking while eating and use smaller plates

Move Your Body Regularly: Engage in regular physical activity, aiming for at least 30 minutes of moderate-intensity exercise most days of the week.

Prioritize Quality Sleep: Aim for 7-8 hours of quality sleep each night. Lack of sleep can disrupt hormones that regulate metabolism and appetite.

By incorporating water into your weight management strategy and adopting a holistic approach that prioritizes healthy living habits, you'll be well on your way to achieving your goals. Remember, consistency is key. Don't be discouraged by setbacks. Celebrate your progress, big or small, and enjoy the journey towards a healthier, happier you.

CHAPTER 7:

GLOWING FROM THE INSIDE OUT: HOW WATER IMPROVES SKIN HEALTH AND APPEARANCE

There is a sure reason for the existence of the term "glowing from the inside out". True beauty transcends superficial layers, reflecting a state of well-being that radiates from within. And one of the most fundamental contributors to this inner glow? Water. In this chapter, we'll delve into the science-backed connection between water and skin health, unveiling how proper hydration can transform your complexion and leave you looking and feeling your best.

Imagine your skin as a magnificent tapestry. Water is the very thread that holds it all together. Here's how:

Hydration Plumps and Fills: Our skin is largely composed of water, around 60% in the outer layer (epidermis). Adequate water intake plumps skin cells, giving your face a youthful, full appearance.

Dehydration, on the other hand, can lead to a dull, sunken look.

Enhanced Elasticity and Flexibility: Water acts as a lubricant between skin cells, keeping them supple and elastic. This translates to a reduction in wrinkles and fine lines, leaving you with a smoother, more youthful appearance.

Aids in Cellular Function: Every process within your skin cells, from collagen production to waste removal, relies on water. Proper hydration ensures these functions operate optimally, promoting healthy cell turnover and a radiant complexion.

Dehydration can manifest on your skin in various ways. Here's how water combats specific concerns:

Dryness and Flaking: When skin lacks moisture, it becomes dry and flaky. Water helps maintain the skin's natural moisture barrier, preventing dryness and promoting a healthy, dewy glow.

Eczema and Psoriasis: While water isn't a cure, studies suggest that proper hydration can improve symptoms of eczema and psoriasis by flushing out toxins and promoting skin barrier function.

Acne Breakouts: Dehydration can trigger your skin to produce excess oil, potentially leading to breakouts. Staying hydrated helps regulate oil production and creates a less hospitable environment for acne-causing bacteria.

Wrinkles and Fine Lines: As mentioned earlier, water plumps skin cells, minimizing the appearance of wrinkles and fine lines. This isn't a magic bullet for eliminating wrinkles, but hydration plays a crucial role in maintaining a youthful appearance.

The benefits of water for your skin extend beyond just keeping it hydrated:

Improved Nutrient Delivery: Water transports essential nutrients throughout your body, including those vital for healthy skin, such as vitamin C, vitamin A, and B vitamins.

Enhanced Blood Flow: Adequate water intake promotes healthy blood circulation, which delivers oxygen and nutrients to your skin cells, promoting a healthy glow.

Waste Removal: Water helps flush toxins and waste products from your body, including those that can contribute to dullness and blemishes.

Unlocking the Power of Water for Radiant Skin

Now that you understand the science, let's explore strategies to unlock the power of water for your skin:

Listen to Your Thirst: While the "eight glasses a day" rule is a general guideline, individual needs vary. Pay attention to your thirst cues – aim for clear urine and avoid feeling excessively thirsty.

Make Water Your Go-To Beverage: Swap sugary drinks and sodas for water. Opt for sparkling water infused with fruits or herbs for a touch of flavor if plain water feels monotonous.

Carry a Reusable Water Bottle: Having a water bottle readily available serves as a constant reminder to sip throughout the day.

Eat Water-Rich Foods: Fruits and vegetables like watermelon, cucumber, and celery have a high water content, contributing to your daily hydration needs.

Monitor Your Skin: Pay attention to how your skin feels and looks. If you notice dryness, flaking, or increased breakouts, it might be a sign you need to increase your water intake.

Start Your Day with Water: Drinking a glass of water first thing in the morning jumpstarts your hydration and metabolism.

Pair Water with Meals and Snacks: Make water your beverage of choice at mealtimes and in between snacks.

Infuse Your Water: Add slices of fruits, herbs, or vegetables to your water for a refreshing and flavorful twist.

Set Hydration Reminders: Use apps or alarms to remind yourself to sip water throughout the day.

Moisturize Regularly: While water hydrates from within, a good moisturizer helps trap moisture in the skin for a dewy, healthy look.

Hydration Beyond Skin Deep: A Holistic Approach for Radiant Beauty

True beauty goes beyond just the surface. While water works wonders for your skin, a holistic approach to hydration brings a symphony of benefits to your overall well-being, further enhancing your inner and outer glow.

Sleep for a Radiant Complexion: During sleep, your skin repairs and regenerates. Adequate sleep (7-8 hours per night) allows these processes to occur optimally, contributing to a radiant complexion. Water plays a crucial role in promoting quality sleep, as dehydration can disrupt sleep patterns.

Stress Management for a Calmer You: Chronic stress can wreak havoc on your skin, leading to breakouts and premature aging. Techniques like meditation, yoga, or deep breathing can help manage stress and promote a calmer state of mind, which can also reflect in a healthier, more relaxed appearance.

A Balanced Diet for Nourished Skin: The old adage "you are what you eat" holds true for your skin as well. A balanced diet rich in fruits, vegetables, whole grains, and lean proteins provides your body with the essential nutrients needed for healthy skin. Water helps transport these nutrients to nourish your cells from within.

Exercise for a Healthy Glow: Regular exercise promotes blood circulation, delivering oxygen and nutrients to your skin cells for a healthy glow. Exercise also helps manage stress and promotes a positive self-image, both of which contribute to inner and outer radiance.

Remember: Consistent hydration is key. Do not stop if you miss a day or two. Focus on developing sustainable habits that work for your lifestyle. Celebrate small victories, and gradually increase your water intake over time.

By embracing the power of water and incorporating these holistic strategies, you'll be well on your way to achieving radiant skin that truly reflects your inner well-being. It's a culmination of healthy habits, a positive mindset, and a state of well-being that shines through. Hydration is a cornerstone of this journey, a simple yet powerful act that can transform your life from the inside out.

So, raise a glass to a future of radiant skin, vibrant health, and a life that glows with the confidence that comes from a body and mind nurtured by the power of water.

STRATEGIES FOR OPTIMAL HYDRATION

CHAPTER 8:

HOW MUCH IS ENOUGH? DETERMINING YOUR INDIVIDUAL WATER NEEDS

Water, the elixir of life, nourishes our bodies, fuels our minds, and plays a vital role in every physiological process. But with the "eight glasses a day" mantra echoing in our ears, a crucial question arises: how much water do I truly need? The answer, like a fingerprint, is uniquely yours.

This chapter delves beyond the one-size-fits-all approach, exploring the factors that influence your individual water needs and equipping you with strategies to embark on your personalized journey to optimal hydration.

Imagine your body as a complex orchestra, with each system an instrument and water acting as the conductor, ensuring all notes are played in harmony. However, the conductor doesn't have a universal volume setting. Several factors act as dials, fine-tuning your body's water requirements:

Body Size: Individuals with larger body size tends to have a greater surface area for evaporation and generate more heat during activity, leading to increased water loss. Think of a large kettle versus a small teapot – both require water, but the kettle needs more to maintain the same level of hydration.

Activity Level: Physical activity, like a vigorous symphony performance, leads to increased sweating. The more active you are, the more water you need to replenish lost fluids and maintain optimal performance.

Climate: Hot and humid environments, like a tropical rainforest, accelerate evaporation and necessitate increased water intake. Conversely, cooler and drier climates may require slightly less water.

Overall Health: Certain medical conditions, like kidney disease or diabetes, can impact your body's ability to regulate fluids. Consulting a healthcare professional for personalized guidance is crucial in these situations.

Diet: A diet rich in fruits and vegetables, akin to a plate overflowing with watermelons and cucumbers, naturally contributes to your hydration needs. Conversely, diets high in processed foods and salty snacks require additional water to flush out excess sodium.

The oft-repeated advice of eight glasses (or 2 liters) of water serves as a reasonable starting point for many healthy adults. However, this is just the first movement in your personalized hydration symphony. Consider these strategies to fine-tune your water intake:

Listen to Your Body's Language: Thirst, the body's built-in dehydration alarm, is a valuable cue. However, don't let it be the sole conductor. Aim to drink water regularly throughout the day, even if you don't feel parched.

Urine, a Window to Hydration: The color of your urine offers a glimpse into your hydration status. Pale yellow indicates adequate hydration, while dark yellow or amber suggests dehydration. Aim for a consistent pale yellow hue.

Track Your Fluid Intake: Become a hydration detective! Keep a log of your water and other fluid intake throughout the day. This self-monitoring helps identify areas for improvement and allows you to adjust your water consumption accordingly.

Technology as Your Hydration Partner: Numerous hydration apps can be your digital allies. These apps let you track your water intake, set personalized reminders based on your activity level and climate, and even offer motivational messages to keep you on track.

Quality Matters: Choosing the Right H2O:

While quantity is essential, the quality of your water also plays a significant role. Here are some considerations:

Filtered Water: Municipal water treatment plants do a great job, but filtering your water at home can further eliminate potential contaminants like chlorine or lead.

Spring Water and Bottled Water: Opt for reputable brands and check the labels for mineral content. While convenient, bottled water can be less eco-friendly than using a reusable water bottle with filtered water.

Making Hydration a Habit: Just like mastering a new instrument takes practice, consistent hydration requires effort. Here are some tips to integrate it seamlessly into your daily routine:

Carry a Reusable Water Bottle: Invest in a reusable water bottle you love and keep it with you throughout the day.

Flavor up Your Water: Plain water can sometimes feel monotonous. Infuse your water with slices of lemon, cucumber, ginger, or mint for a refreshing twist.

Embrace Water-Rich Foods: Fruits and vegetables, nature's water bombs, are a delicious way to boost your hydration. Integrate them generously into your meals and snacks.

Pair Water with Activities: Develop a habit of drinking water before, during, and after exercise. Similarly, link water consumption with other daily routines, like taking a shower or checking your email.

Remember, the ultimate goal is to feel your best. Here are some additional signs that you might be dehydrated, even if you're not experiencing intense thirst:

Fatigue and Lack of Energy: Dehydration can zap your energy levels, making you feel sluggish and tired.

Headaches: Dehydration is a common culprit behind headaches. Proper hydration can help prevent or alleviate them.

Difficulty Concentrating: Dehydration can impair cognitive function, making it harder to focus and concentrate.

Dry Mouth and Skin: Dryness in your mouth and on your skin can be indicators of dehydration.

Constipation: Water plays a crucial role in digestion. Constipation and other digestive problems can be as a result of Dehydration.

Reduced Exercise Performance: Feeling tired, sluggish, or experiencing muscle cramps during exercise can be signs of dehydration.

Understanding these signs can help you stay ahead of dehydration and ensure you're operating at peak capacity.

The Power of Habit: Building a Sustainable Hydration Routine

Building a sustainable hydration routine requires integrating small, achievable practices into your daily life. Here are some strategies:

Set Realistic Goals: Don't try to go from zero to eight glasses overnight. Start with small, incremental increases and gradually build your water intake over time.

Pair Water with Meals and Snacks: Make it a habit to drink a glass of water before, during, and after meals and snacks. This helps with digestion and ensures you're getting enough fluids throughout the day.

Plan for Social Gatherings: Social events can sometimes lead to neglecting water intake. Bring your reusable water bottle or plan to order water throughout the gathering.

Reward Yourself: Celebrate your progress! Reaching your daily hydration goals or completing a hydration challenge deserves a reward. Choose a non-food reward, like a relaxing bath or a new book.

Hydration Hacks for Different Lifestyles:

For the Busy Professional: Keep a water bottle at your desk and set reminders on your computer or phone to prompt you to drink water throughout the day.

For Travelers: Be mindful of potential dehydration risks in unfamiliar environments, especially in hot climates. Go along with your reusable water bottle and refill it once empty.

For Pregnant and Breastfeeding Women: Increased water needs are crucial during pregnancy and breastfeeding.

For Older Adults: As we age, thirst perception can diminish. Make a conscious effort to stay hydrated, even if you don't feel particularly thirsty.

By incorporating these tips and tailoring them to your individual needs, you can create a sustainable hydration routine that supports your overall well-being.

Water is the foundation of life, the conductor of your internal orchestra. By understanding your individual needs, employing these strategies, and making hydration a priority, you can unlock a symphony of well-being within you. Remember, consistency is key. Celebrate your progress, big or small, and enjoy the vibrant melody of a well-hydrated life!

CHAPTER 9:

BEYOND PLAIN WATER: FLAVORFUL AND FUNCTIONAL HYDRATION

(Options 110. Making it a habit: tips and tricks for consistent water consumption)

While plain water remains the cornerstone of optimal hydration, sometimes we crave a little more pizazz. This chapter explores a world of flavorful and functional options to keep your taste buds happy and your hydration on track.

Let's face it, plain water, while essential, can sometimes feel monotonous. Here's where your inner mixologist can come alive! Explore these natural flavor enhancers to transform your water from ordinary to extraordinary:

Citrus Symphony: A splash of lemon, lime, orange, or grapefruit adds a refreshing zing to your water. Experiment with different combinations to create your perfect citrusy blend.

Berry Blast: Muddle fresh or frozen berries like strawberries, blueberries, or raspberries into your water for a burst of sweetness and antioxidants.

Stone Fruit Splash: Thinly sliced peaches, nectarines, or plums add a touch of sweetness and a subtle summery flavor to your water.

Herbal Haven: Fresh herbs like mint, basil, or rosemary can infuse your water with a unique and invigorating flavor.

Spice up Your Life: For a warm and comforting touch, consider adding a sliver of ginger or a pinch of cinnamon to your water. These spices also have potential health benefits.

Cucumber Coolness: Sliced cucumber adds a refreshing and slightly sweet flavor to your water, making it perfect for a hot summer day.

Looking for a little extra functionality with your hydration? Explore these options:

Sparkling Water: For a bubbly twist, opt for unsweetened sparkling water. While not a replacement for plain water due to its carbonation, it can be a refreshing alternative in moderation.

Coconut Water: A natural source of electrolytes like potassium, magnesium, and sodium, coconut water can be a good choice for replenishing fluids after exercise or on a hot day. However, be mindful of the sugar content in some commercially available brands.

Fruit-Infused Waters: Commercially available fruit-infused waters can be a convenient option, but be sure to check the label for added sugars and artificial ingredients. Opt for natural options whenever possible.

A Note on Sweeteners: While adding a squeeze of natural fruit juice or a few drops of stevia can be acceptable in moderation, it's important to limit added sugars in your water. Excessive sugar intake can contribute to various health problems, negating the benefits of hydration.

Experimentation is Key:

The beauty of these choices lies in their versatility. Explore different combinations to discover your favorites. Remember, the key is to find flavors and functionalities that encourage you to drink more water throughout the day.

Safety Considerations: Certain fruits, like grapefruit, can interact with medications. If you have any concerns, consult your healthcare professional before adding them to your water.

Making It Fun for Everyone: Getting the whole family involved in flavorful hydration can be a fun and healthy endeavor. Here are some ideas:

Host a "Flavor Fusion" party: Let everyone experiment with different flavor combinations and create their signature infused water recipes.

Involve the kids in the preparation: Engaging children in slicing fruits or herbs for their water can make them more invested in staying hydrated.

Get creative with containers: Invest in fun and colorful reusable water bottles for the whole family to make hydration visually appealing.

By incorporating these flavorful and functional options, you can transform water from a chore into a delightful and healthy habit.

Making it a Habit: Tips and Tricks for Consistent Water Consumption

We've explored the importance of hydration, the factors influencing individual needs, and the world of flavorful options to elevate your water experience. Now comes the crucial part: building consistent hydration habits that ensure you're reaping the benefits of water every day.

Let's be honest, remembering to drink water consistently can be a challenge. Here are some strategies to combat forgetfulness and make hydration a seamless part of your routine:

Invest in a Reusable Water Bottle: Find a reusable water bottle you love, one that fits your style and is convenient to carry around. Carry along with you always serves as a constant reminder to sip throughout the day.

The Power of Apps: Download a hydration app! These apps can be your digital hydration coaches, sending reminders, tracking your water intake, and even offering motivational messages to keep you on track.

Pair Water with Activities: Develop the habit of drinking water before, during, and after specific activities. For example, make water your go-to beverage every time you wake up, before and after meals, and before, during, and after exercise.

Utilize Technology: Many smartphones and smart watches come with built-in water tracking features or allow integration with hydration apps. Utilize these features to set reminders and monitor your progress.

Strategic Placement: Keep a reusable water bottle filled with water on your desk, in your car, and at strategic locations around your house. This constant visual cue will prompt you to take a sip.

Habits are formed through repetition and positive reinforcement. Here's how to apply this concept to hydration:

The Cue: Identify cues that trigger you to drink something. It could be feeling thirsty, waking up, or finishing a meal.

The Craving: Associate the cue with the positive feeling of refreshing, hydrating water.

The Response: Make grabbing your water bottle your automatic response to the cue.

The Reward: Celebrate your progress! Completing a hydration challenge or reaching your daily water goal can be rewarded with a non-food treat, like a relaxing bath or a new book.

Life throws different curveballs our way. Here are some tips to maintain hydration in various situations:

At Work: Keep your reusable water bottle filled at your desk and set reminders on your computer or phone to prompt you to drink water regularly.

On the Go: Invest in a good quality insulated water bottle that keeps your water cold throughout the day, especially during travel or commutes.

During Social Gatherings: Social settings can sometimes lead to neglecting water intake. Bring your reusable water bottle or plan to order water throughout the event.

While Traveling: Be mindful of potential dehydration risks in unfamiliar environments, especially in hot climates.

Hydration for Special Needs:

Pregnant and Breastfeeding Women: Increased water needs are crucial during pregnancy and breastfeeding. Consult your healthcare professional for personalized guidance on how much water you should be drinking.

Older Adults: As we age, thirst perception can diminish. Make a conscious effort to stay hydrated, even if you don't feel particularly thirsty.

Embrace the Power of Community: Staying accountable can be easier with a support system. Share your Experience with friends and family. Encourage each other and celebrate milestones together. You can also join online hydration communities for motivation and inspiration.

Remember, consistency is key. Do not stop if you miss a day or two. The goal is to develop sustainable habits that fit your lifestyle. Start small, celebrate progress, and gradually increase your water intake over time.

By incorporating these tips and tricks, you can transform water from a simple drink into a cornerstone of your health and well-being. Enjoy the process, explore the flavorful options, and celebrate the vibrant life that flourishes with every sip!

CHAPTER 10:

OVER HYDRATION: UNDERSTANDING THE RISKS AND FINDING BALANCE

While we've established the importance of staying hydrated, it's crucial to acknowledge that too much of a good thing can sometimes be detrimental. This chapter explores the potential risks of over hydration and guides you towards finding the perfect balance for optimal health.

Over hydration occurs when you consume fluids, primarily water, faster than your kidneys can eliminate them. While rare, it can lead to an electrolyte imbalance in the bloodstream, a condition known as electrolyte imbalance or hyponatremia. Electrolytes are minerals like sodium, potassium, and chloride that play essential roles in various bodily functions, including muscle function, nerve transmission, and maintaining blood pressure.

Factors Contributing to Over Hydration:

Several factors can put you at an increased risk of over hydration:

Excessive Water Consumption: While exceeding the recommended daily intake occasionally might not pose a significant risk, consistently consuming large amounts of water, particularly in a short period, can lead to over hydration.

Underlying Medical Conditions: Certain medical conditions, such as heart failure, kidney disease, or liver disease, can affect your body's ability to regulate fluids and electrolyte balance.

Medications: Diuretics, which are medications used to treat high blood pressure or certain heart conditions, can increase urine output and potentially contribute to over hydration if excessive fluids are consumed.

Endurance Events: Athletes participating in prolonged endurance events, especially in hot and humid environments, are at increased risk of over hydration if they solely focus on water intake without considering electrolyte replacement.

Signs and Symptoms of Over hydration:

While thirst is a natural indicator of dehydration, excessive thirst can also be a sign of over hydration. Here are some symptoms to look out for:

Headaches: Headaches are a common symptom of electrolyte imbalance caused by over hydration.

Nausea and Vomiting: Over hydration can trigger nausea and vomiting as your body attempts to expel excess fluids.

Confusion and Disorientation: Severe over hydration can lead to confusion, disorientation, and even seizures.

Muscle Weakness and Cramps: Electrolyte imbalance can disrupt muscle function, leading to weakness and cramps.

Fatigue and Lethargy: Over hydration can cause feelings of fatigue and sluggishness.

Seizures: In extreme cases of over hydration, especially in individuals with underlying medical conditions, seizures can occur.

Early detection of over hydration is crucial to prevent complications. If you experience any of the symptoms mentioned above, particularly after consuming large amounts of water, it's essential to seek medical attention immediately.

Finding the Balance: Personalized Hydration Strategies

The key to optimal hydration lies in finding the balance that works for your unique body. Here are some strategies to ensure you're getting enough water without going overboard:

Listen to Your Body: Thirst is a valuable indicator. Drink water throughout the day, even if you don't feel intensely thirsty, but avoid forcing fluids down if you're not feeling parched.

Monitor Your Urine Color: Pale yellow urine generally indicates good hydration, while dark yellow or amber urine suggests dehydration. Aim for a consistent pale yellow hue.

Consider Individual Needs: Factors like activity level, climate, and overall health influence your water needs. Tailor your water intake accordingly. Consulting a healthcare professional can help you determine the optimal amount of water for your specific situation.

Focus on Electrolytes for Endurance Activities: Athletes participating in extended exercise, especially in hot weather, should prioritize electrolyte replacement alongside adequate water intake. Consult a nutritionist or sports physician for personalized guidance on electrolyte needs.

Food as a Source of Hydration: Remember, water isn't the only source of hydration. Many fruits and vegetables have a high water content and can contribute to your daily fluid intake.

Technology Can Be Your Ally: Hydration apps can be valuable tools, but it's important to use them as a guide, not a rigid rule. These apps can offer personalized hydration recommendations based on your activity level and climate, but always prioritize your body's signals over app suggestions.

The Importance of Individualized Medical Advice: While this chapter provides general information, it's not a substitute for professional medical advice. Individuals with underlying health conditions or concerns about over hydration should consult a healthcare professional for personalized guidance.

While water remains the cornerstone of optimal hydration, a holistic approach that considers other factors can further enhance your well-being:

Electrolyte Balance: Consuming electrolyte-rich foods like fruits, vegetables, and dairy products can help maintain electrolyte balance, especially for individuals at risk of over hydration.

Electrolyte Supplements: In certain situations, such as during extended endurance events or for individuals with specific medical conditions, electrolyte supplements may be recommended by a healthcare professional. However, it's crucial to avoid self-prescribing electrolyte supplements, as excessive intake can also be detrimental.

Sleep: Adequate sleep plays a vital role in regulating fluid balance. Aim for 7-8 hours of quality sleep each night to support optimal hydration.

Stress Management: Chronic stress can disrupt various bodily functions, including fluid regulation. Techniques like meditation, yoga, or deep breathing can help manage stress and promote a healthy hydration balance.

Finding the perfect hydration balance is an ongoing journey, a beautiful symphony where you listen to your body's unique cues and adjust your strategies accordingly. Remember, consistency is key. Celebrate your progress, big or small, and embrace the vibrant life that flourishes with a balanced approach to hydration.

Additional Considerations:

Environmental Conditions: Be mindful of your environment. Hot and humid climates or high-altitude settings can increase your water needs. Adjust your intake accordingly.

Dietary Choices: A diet high in processed foods or diuretics like caffeine can necessitate increased water intake to compensate for fluid loss.

Age: As we age, thirst perception can diminish. Make a conscious effort to stay hydrated, even if you don't feel particularly thirsty.

Building a Sustainable Hydration Routine:

Set Realistic Goals: Don't aim for drastic changes overnight. Start with small, achievable goals and gradually increase your water intake over time.

Make it a Habit: Make drinking Water your daily routine. Pair water with meals and snacks, set reminders on your phone, or find an activity buddy who can support your hydration journey.

Celebrate Milestones: Reward yourself for reaching your hydration goals. This can help maintain motivation and make hydration a more enjoyable experience.

By incorporating these strategies and finding your personal hydration sweet spot, you can unlock a world of optimal health and well-being. Remember, water is the conductor of your internal orchestra. Listen to its subtle cues, find the right balance, and experience the beautiful melody of a life vibrantly hydrated!

CHAPTER 11:

HYDRATION FOR LIFE STAGES: TAILORING WATER INTAKE FOR CHILDREN, ADULTS, AND SENIORS

Water, the elixir of life, plays a crucial role throughout our lifespan. However, hydration needs can vary significantly depending on our age and stage of development. This chapter delves into the unique hydration requirements of children, adults, and seniors, equipping you with the knowledge to tailor water intake for optimal health across all life stages.

Hydration Heroes: Ensuring Optimal Water Intake for Children

Children are like little sponges, constantly growing and developing. Proper hydration is essential for their physical and cognitive well-being. Here's a closer look at the hydration needs of children at different stages:

Infants (0-12 months): Breast milk or formula is the primary source of fluids for infants. However, in hot weather or during illness, additional water or an electrolyte solution may be recommended by a pediatrician.

Toddlers (1-3 years): Toddlers are busy explorers, and their thirst perception might not be fully developed. Offer water frequently throughout the day, even if they don't ask for it. Opt for spill-proof sippy cups and make water breaks a fun part of their routine.

Preschoolers (4-6 years): Preschoolers are becoming more active and independent. Encourage them to carry a reusable water bottle and take regular sips. Incorporate water into mealtimes and snack breaks.

School-Aged Children (6-12 years): School activities and outdoor play increase water needs. Pack a reusable water bottle for school and encourage them to drink throughout the day. Sports practices and games necessitate additional water intake to replenish fluids lost through sweat.

Tips for Encouraging Hydration in Children:

Make it Fun: Use colorful and attractive water bottles with their favorite characters.

Lead by Example: Let your children see you drinking water regularly.

Incorporate Flavor: Add slices of fruits like cucumber, lemon, or berries to their water for a refreshing twist.

Freeze Fun: Freeze water balloons or fruit-infused ice pops for a cool and hydrating treat.

Reward Good Habits: Celebrate their progress in developing healthy hydration habits.

Hydration Champions: Maintaining Optimal Hydration throughout Adulthood

As adults, our water needs can vary based on several factors like activity level, climate, and overall health. Here's a breakdown of considerations for adults:

Active Adults: Physical activity increases sweat production and fluid loss. Increase water intake before, during, and after exercise to stay hydrated.

Consider electrolyte-rich beverages for extended or intense workouts.

Pregnant and Breastfeeding Women: Increased water needs are crucial during pregnancy and breastfeeding. Consult a healthcare professional for personalized guidance on optimal water intake.

Travelers: Be mindful of potential dehydration risks in unfamiliar environments, especially in hot climates. Travel along with water bottle and refill it frequently.

Individuals with Medical Conditions: Certain medical conditions can affect your fluid balance. Consult a healthcare professional for personalized hydration advice if you have any concerns.

Strategies for Consistent Hydration in Adults:

Invest in a Reusable Water Bottle: Carry a water bottle you love and keep it with you throughout the day.

Download a Hydration App: Use hydration apps to track your water intake, set reminders, and stay motivated.

Pair Water with Activities: Develop the habit of drinking water before, during, and after meals and snacks.

Strategically Place Water Bottles: Keep a water bottle at your desk, in your car, and at various locations around your house for easy access.

Make Water Flavorful: Infuse your water with fruits, herbs, or spices for a refreshing twist.

Hydration Guardians: Ensuring Proper Hydration for Seniors

As we age, thirst perception can diminish, and our bodies become less efficient at regulating fluids. Here's how to ensure proper hydration for seniors:

Set Reminders: Schedule alarms or use reminder apps to prompt regular water intake throughout the day.

Choose Easy-to-Grip Water Bottles: Opt for water bottles with easy-to-grip handles to prevent spills and ensure accessibility.

Incorporate Water-Rich Foods: Fruits and vegetables with high water content, like watermelon, celery, and cucumber, can contribute to hydration.

Monitor Urine Color: Pale yellow urine indicates adequate hydration, while dark yellow urine suggests dehydration. Encourage seniors to report any changes in urine color to their healthcare professional.

Medical Supervision: For seniors with underlying health conditions, healthcare professionals can provide personalized guidance on water intake and monitor their hydration status.

Additional Considerations for Seniors:

Medications: Certain medications can be diuretics, increasing urine output. Consult a healthcare professional to determine if medication adjustments or increased water intake are necessary to maintain proper hydration.

Cognitive Decline: In cases of dementia or other cognitive decline, ensuring proper hydration can become challenging. Family caregivers may need to take on a more active role in reminding and assisting seniors with drinking water.

Limited Mobility: Reduced mobility can make accessing water more difficult. Ensure seniors have readily available water bottles within easy reach and offer assistance if needed.

Building a Culture of Hydration for All Ages

Hydration is a lifelong journey. By fostering a culture of hydration within families and communities, we can ensure everyone, regardless of age, thrives with a healthy water balance. Here's how:

Lead by Example: Adults can set a positive example for children by prioritizing their own hydration and encouraging healthy water habits.

Incorporate Water into Family Meals and Activities: Make water the default beverage during mealtimes and encourage family outings to involve water breaks.

Educate Children on the Importance of Hydration: Teach children about the benefits of water for their health and well-being, using age-appropriate language and fun visuals.

Advocate for Hydration in Schools and Communities: Support initiatives that promote hydration in schools and community centers. This could involve installing water fountains, offering educational programs, or organizing hydration challenges.

Hydration needs may evolve throughout our life stages, but its importance remains constant. By understanding and addressing the unique hydration requirements of each age group, we can orchestrate a symphony of well-being that resonates throughout life. Remember, consistency is key. Celebrate progress, big or small, and cultivate a lifelong love affair with water – the elixir of life for every stage of your journey.

This chapter equips you with the knowledge to tailor water intake for optimal health across all life stages. Remember, water is the conductor of your internal orchestra at every age. Listen to its subtle cues, find the right balance, and experience the beautiful melody of a life vibrantly hydrated!

CONCLUSION

This journey through the science of water has unveiled its profound impact on our physical and mental well-being. You've now discovered how water plays a vital role in every system within us, from boosting energy to sharpening focus.

Remember, consistent hydration is not a destination, but a ripple effect that spreads throughout your life. By incorporating the strategies you've learned, you can create a sustainable hydration routine, empowering your body and mind to thrive.

So raise a glass (or reusable water bottle!) to the simple yet powerful act of drinking water. May every sip be a step towards a healthier, happier you!